HEALING YOUR BACK OF CHRONIC PAIN

REVERSING HABITUAL RESPONSES

Dr. Christopher Maloney, N.D.

ISBN-13: 978-1976214974
ISBN-10: 1976214971

DEDICATION

For all those patients who taught me about their pain.
May you all be well and thank you.

CONTENTS

ACKNOWLEDGMENTS

I want to thank the tireless researchers who provide us with answers about our bodies. Thank you to Joe, my proofreader, business partner, and friend. Thank you to R, A, E, G, and my other patients who have read and commented on the book. I do listen and try to improve. To my family, my eternal thanks for bearing with me as I pour over medical texts. To my colleagues and teachers, you have taught me more than I can remember. And thank you, dear reader, for taking the time to care enough about your own back.

WARNING

This book is for informational purposes and is not intended as a substitute for the medical advice of physicians. The reader should consult a physician if they have any symptoms that may require diagnosis or medical attention. Be wise and take care of yourselves!

1 WHY THIS BOOK?

Congratulations on starting your journey away from chronic pain. Every journey begins with a single step, and you've taken that step by looking for this book and finding it. If you have chronic back pain, then this book is for you. It may help when nothing else has.

To be clear, nothing in this book replaces common sense. If you are in a car accident, please do not haul this book out of the crushed glove compartment and expect it to replace surgery. Get yourself patched up, and read this book only after your surgeons have stabilized your spine.

But if you've had multiple surgeries without success, then this book may be more helpful than one more surgery. Most surgeons know there is a decreasing return after initial surgeries, and will do additional surgeries reluctantly.

Many books on back pain focus entirely on exercise routines. So I assume you have access to those and may have tried some already. If you haven't, some of you may benefit from learning how to stretch the muscles of the back.

Instead of another physical treatment or set of exercises, we will talk in this book about habitual responses in the back. We will look at how habitual responses can trigger chronic muscle tension in the back, leading to pain. These responses may be to a physical cause, but they may also be generated by an emotional state or even by mental stress that leads to physical tension in the back. By helping you recognize these responses, we may completely resolve chronic back pain that has not been helped by other treatments.

We're talking specifically about back pain that has continued despite drugs and treatment, especially if you have more pain when you're stressed. If you've read psychology books on letting go of stress, you may have tried to resolve your pain by telling yourself it is strictly mental. One famous back doctor has had some success with this mental model. But the mental model denies the reality that many pains worsened by stress also have physical triggers that are not under our conscious control. The conscious mind can work through the stresses you are aware of, releasing that tension. But unconscious, habitual stress may escape notice or be retriggered by movement, by familiar situations, or by simply having a similar emotional feeling.

For those of you who have doubts that anything will help your chronic back pain, let me tell you a story.

When she was young, Jane (not her real name) was in a terrible car accident. After mostly healing from the accident, Jane found herself still suffering with chronic back pain. It wasn't quite bad enough for additional surgery, so she was sent out from the hospital with debilitating, agonizing pain. By the time she found me twenty years later, she'd been to every back specialist under the sun and had nothing to show for it except an addiction to painkillers.

The painkillers did help Jane with her pain, but they weren't enough. She was on eight Oxycontin a day, the maximum her doctor would prescribe. Despite the drugs, she lived her life in a fog of pain. Before the accident, Jane had been thinking about college, maybe even becoming a doctor. But after the accident, she couldn't focus. She had dropped out of college, married, and had children. So to the outside world she was coping with her pain. But every day she had to make a list of the things she was supposed to do, double check that she turned off the stove, and live in constant fear that she might forget to pick up one of her kids from school.

When I saw Jane, she was at the end of her rope. Conventional options had been exhausted long ago. She had heard about me from another patient, but was highly skeptical that anything we could do would help her. I looked at her lab reports, X-rays, and CT scan. Nothing in them showed any reason for her pain. Certainly nothing to justify a surgery.

So then I did something that most of her doctors had not done. I examined her back in detail with my hands.

Jane's whole back was a board, no flexibility anywhere. Imagine tensing your entire back, every muscle, and holding that tension all day and all night. That was her normal back tension. Of course that would hurt! Part of her pain was simply from muscle exhaustion.

As the back muscles tire, they switch from using oxygen to help burn sugar for energy to burning sugar without oxygen. Like a fire in the fireplace, the lack of oxygen means that the muscles burn less efficiently and that causes them to build up acid. The acid hurts if there's too much of it in a muscle. The pain sensation you get in your arm from trying to hold a weight up for too long is from too much acid (metabolic acidosis). Jane's entire back under constant tension burned like that all the time.

As we worked on Jane's back together, she gradually released. Just feeling the release was enough to bring some tears of relief. Many of my patients no longer believe any relief is possible, so it can be emotional to hope for improvement again.

After several visits the back was mostly relaxed. We found one bone in the middle of her back that would pop out of place. It would happen every time she lifted anything or every time she felt stressed about her children. When her back went out of place, her muscles would spasm over the entire back to protect it from further damage just as they had after the original car accident so many years before. It was the root cause of the pain.

Unraveling Jane's specific pain and its triggers was the curative treatment, though it took some time to figure out everything that triggered her. After our work together, she was able to decrease her Oxycontin doses and eventually went off all medication. I haven't seen her in some years now. At times her pain returns, but she's able to deal with it without drugs. Her life didn't become perfect, but she doesn't have the pain she had before. By working with her body rather than trying to ignore it, she has found a path to relief.

Many doctors who work with chronic pain want to see you all the time. They need to treat you multiple times a week forever for the treatment to work. My best patients are those who I see for a period of months who learn how to heal themselves. I don't need to see them again for years at a time, because they are able to resolve their own pain. These are determined people who have continued to pursue their paths to health long after others would have accepted pain as a daily companion. Together we've worked to find what works for them on a daily basis. I hope to give you the tools we've developed together, to help you understand and heal your pain.

2 BORN TO PAIN

Just now, as I tilted myself in my chair, I felt three different pops in my upper back. It's not uncommon for me to need to shift myself to let go of tension and pain a dozen or more times a day.

When I was twelve an enterprising chiropractor examined me and found a goldmine. My left side is shorter than my right, and my torso shows lowered ribs on the left side. He sold me a lift for my left foot, and prescribed weekly treatments for the rest of my life. If that wasn't enough, I also had lordosis, an overly curved lower spine. My chiropractor told me it was due to weak stomach muscles, leading to hundreds of sweaty sit ups for years afterward. Add to that a compressed spinal fracture from high school, and there is no reason to think I wouldn't live my life in pain or sucking down painkillers.

But I don't. As I'm writing, I don't experience pain.

It isn't because of my perpetual ongoing treatments. Within a few months I'd stopped chiropractic because it didn't help me much. I stopped the sit ups a bit later after straining my stomach muscles. In college, I finally dumped the lift for my left foot because it annoyed me and never looked back. Currently my back pain is managed by me and an occasional gentle massage.

Not that shoveling snow or overdoing running doesn't cause me pain. I encounter pain and resolve it. It doesn't linger or set up permanently in my body, because I use a wide variety of techniques to move beyond it.

My experience is not uncommon. Over the last two decades I've seen hundreds of backs. I've never seen a perfect spine, nor a perfect body. We all have our oddities that could explain any amount of pain. But one of the unspoken miracles of medicine is the number of people who "should" experience pain but don't. On the other side is the nightmare of people who should be fine because there's nothing visibly wrong with them, but they are in agony.

In my radiology class, reading X-rays and CT scans, I remember looking at "normal" spines from patients without pain. Some of them had horrible breaks, poorly healed and teetering precariously on top of other bones like a tower about to fall. But they had no symptoms, no pain. Other patients showed me beautiful, nearly perfect X-rayed spines while they writhed in agony on the examination table. If the physical changes in the spine don't determine physical pain levels, what does?

Treating myself for pain led to an interest in the pain of others. I moved from learning massage to going to premedical studies. When I looked at medical schools, I decided to attend a Naturopathic Medical School because that license would give me more freedom to explore both the causes and possible treatments for chronic pain.

I've spent the last dozen years working with patients who have taught me about their pain. What they've shown me is that the pain they feel is not in their heads, it's in their backs. But that doesn't mean it isn't profoundly influenced by their habitual attitudes and responses toward that pain.

3 NOT GETTING BETTER ON ITS OWN

One of the classic lies people with chronic back pain tell themselves is that their backs will improve with time. Many studies report that those suffering from back pain return to work or stop consulting their doctors after about a month. But follow-up studies show over half of those people continue to experience significant back pain.[i] So the patients are considered successes by the medical profession because they are back at work, but every day they are limited by pain that remains as their constant companion.

So what does happen over time with a chronic back problem? What increases with time is scarring, which tightens your back and can increase pain. Muscle tension also increases over time, which can cause your bones to lay down calcium deposits at areas of great tension. The

X-rays pick up the calcium deposits, leading to diagnoses of bone spurs or degenerative joint disease in the areas of high tension. Once you have a bone diagnosis, chances are you will only get pain medication until the situation becomes bad enough to justify surgery.

But people with chronic back pain do remember that the pain was different or better in the past. As the years pass, many patients underestimate how much pain they were in before.[ii] They'll tell their doctors they only had a three or four pain on a ten point scale before, when the older records show that they reported an eight or a nine. So their memory of past pain fades in proportion to their current pain.[iii] The pain doesn't.

It can be protective of your sanity to pretend your pain wasn't always this bad. If you've been to a specialist who has looked at your back and doesn't think you're a candidate for surgery, all you may be given is a prescription painkiller. Then you're told to go home and "live with it." Part of living with it is downplaying how much it hurts every day. You focus your life on getting through today, narrowing your focus and your willpower on overcoming today's pain. No wonder yesterday's pain seems less, and your pain from ten years ago is a distant, faint memory.

If you've managed to tolerate your pain, and deal with

your pain on a daily basis in part by ignoring it, it can be very scary to face your pain fully again. Sometimes taking a long look at your life and the next ten years is not something you want to do when you're struggling with today's crises. So if you find yourself today unable to cope, read on but promise yourself that you'll be gentle and take things at your own pace.

If you're fed-up with the pain, and no longer want it to be the same tomorrow, then we need to work together today to lessen it. If you have been down this path before, you know that facing your pain can make it seem worse. Suddenly you're aware of every twinge, every spasm. Even as I'm writing I can feel tension creeping up the right side of my neck. The awareness of pain can make it loom as large as a charging bull in our vision. But only by facing the bull can we ever hope to heal it.

4 PHYSICAL TREATMENTS THAT WORK

As I was writing this book, the American College of Physicians came out with a new set of guidelines on using opiates for back pain.[iv] After decades of piling on the drugs, the new standard is "just say no." They no longer recommend opiates for back pain. That's right, it's back to the lesser pain medications. Why? Because there is little evidence that the opiates help more, and good evidence that they are more addictive.

It's hard to understand just how big this shift is until you realize that opiates are the number one drug prescription in my state. They are overwhelmingly prescribed for pain, and nationwide back pain accounts for the majority of pain diagnoses. So we're talking about a huge shift; moving patients off opiates and onto...what?

The other common pain drugs, the nonsteroidal anti-inflammatory drugs (NSAIDS) like Advil or Tylenol, help a little with the pain. But presumably the reason people prefer the opiates is because they are better at helping with the pain. Another study came out recently saying that only one in six people taking NSAID drugs felt any benefit over placebo. [v] That leaves five of every six, about 80%, of chronic pain sufferers still suffering while taking NSAIDs.

When eighty percent of people with chronic back pain aren't getting relief, they want some alternatives. And if opiates are no longer on the menu, what else is there? Is there good evidence that other things help more than NSAIDs with chronic back pain? Yes and no.

No One Truly Knows What Works.

Let's start by saying no one really knows for sure what will help, or what will help most with chronic back pain. Not your wise family doctor and not even an elite Ivy League back surgeon specializing in chronic back pain. Why? Because we have no standard tool for measuring back pain despite decades of pleas by doctors to come up with one standard.[vi]

Today doctors are using sixty-six different measuring tools for pain and forty-four different measurements for disability. When you compare the different measuring tools to see if they are measuring the same things, they overlap only about ten percent of the time. [vii] So one study on chronic back pain could say a treatment works, while another study using another measuring test says it doesn't work. Both can be right, because they're using different ways of measuring.

But surely some things work regardless of the measuring tool? If the tide is coming in, it doesn't matter which ruler you use to measure it. All of them will show that the beach is getting smaller. Are there treatments for chronic back pain that consistently show improvements across all the studies and measuring tests? No.

Surgery

You'd think back surgery would always work. Seriously. If I go in and saw away the bone around your pinched nerve, shouldn't that nerve take a long, deep sigh, and stop hurting? But that's not what we see. Back surgery often doesn't do what it's supposed to do for chronic back pain.

If you're in a massive trauma, like skydiving without a parachute, ignore me and get yourself patched up with all the surgery you need. I'm talking to the people who've been patched up, given the "go home and live with it" prescription, and still can't get through the day without lying on the floor moaning. These are the people who may not find relief from more surgery.

One standard type of surgery for chronic back pain has been spinal fusion. If that bone is hurting you, we'll screw it or glue it to the nearby bones so it doesn't move anymore. It sounds good until you start thinking about the nearby bones, which now need to take on extra load and movement. I've seen patients need one fusion after another. The current record I've seen personally is twelve fusions, each necessary because the previous fusion made the next joint of the spine unstable. At last the poor man gave up on surgery as a solution for his chronic pain. The medical research experts agree. A review of all the fusion studies now says that spinal fusion should no longer be used for chronic low back pain. [viii]

But that doesn't mean spinal fusion isn't still being done or recommended to patients. There tends to be a ten-year delay from the time research comes out to the time doctors change their habits. Doctors are like anyone else; they don't like to change what they're doing, and they don't tend to trust new studies that say they're wrong.

But what about the most popular surgery for chronic back pain, a discectomy? A discectomy is cutting out the padding discs between the bones of a person's back. With trauma or constant use, the fluid discs between the back's boney vertebrae can tear and rupture, giving a clear X-ray reason to do surgery. Disc hurting? Take out the disc. No disc, no pain. Does it work? For a little while.

In the first few months, people in chronic pain felt better without their discs. [ix] But that improvement didn't last for many patients. After about two years it was hard to tell in many patients who got the disc surgery and who did not based on pain levels.[x] Except the patients who'd had the surgery had more complications than those who did not. They spent more time in the hospital and needed more medical care.

In response to the poor outcomes from full disc removal, a newer, less intrusive surgery is being tried. It just removes the little fragments of the torn disc without taking out the whole disc. So far, the little fragment removal gets about the same result as the full disc removal.[xi] In other words, short term relief, but with decreasing results over time.

Chiropractic

If not surgery, you'd think that chiropractic adjustments would always work. Again, you've got a bone out of place in your back, pinching a nerve, and the chiropractor pushes it back in place. Shouldn't the nerve heave a sigh of relief? But, over time, chiropractic works about as well as other physical treatments for chronic back pain. It's helpful short-term but not long-term. [xii]

If you're like me, the chiropractic pop lasts all of twenty minutes. By the time you're walking out the door, you can already feel the bone edging its way out of place. That doesn't mean that chiropractic isn't helpful for sudden minor trauma. When I do something that puts my ribs or neck out, having someone pop me back into place is great.

Patients also tend to prefer chiropractors because they communicate more with patients, taking more time than most MDs.[xiii] Individual results may vary, as they do with MDs and DCs. Good caregivers are wonderful, and short-term relief is much better than none. So by all means continue any care that is helping, just don't expect it to resolve all your pain over the long term.

Massage

My personal preference is for massage over chiropractic, and studies say it may or may not be as effective. One study I found puts the effect of a good massage at longer than a year. Other studies found no long term effect.[xiv] Many back pain sufferers have experienced a range of different treatments, and should definitely add massage to other bodywork as a possibility for short term relief.

Other Physical Body Workers

We could go on: Osteopaths, Physical Therapists, Occupational Therapists, Ergonomic Specialists, Rolfers, and Sports Teachers, can all be effective short-term for back pain. They may use any number of physical treatments, including acupuncture, various massage machines, stretches, ointments and lifestyle changes.

All these interventions may be helpful short-term, less so long-term. Purely physical interventions all work primarily on rearranging the muscles around the nerve, and that relief tends to be temporary. But temporary relief is still far better than no relief.

Cutting Nerves

But what about intense, last-ditch interventions? Forget disc surgery. Who hasn't wanted at times to just have them inject that nerve and kill it? Or cut it out? And here we should see a definite, conclusive long-term result.

Right?

If I go into your back and inject your nerve with an anesthetic that tells it to stop hurting, then we would assume that would take care of your back pain. Injecting a painful nerve with an anesthetic did help prevent the need for surgery, but only short term. Long term, people still got surgery at about the same rate. [xv]

Forget injections. Just cut the nerve! Cutting the nerve - denervation - would seem to be the ultimate pain-ending solution. Except when it's not.

While cutting the nerve was slightly better at pain relief than injecting it, and the short-term results were good, over the long term the pain relief results were small for some kinds of back pain and non-existent for others. [xvi] How is this possible? Nerves regrow, reconnect, or the body finds another route to bring feeling back to the area. Some patients even experience phantom pain, like they might after the loss of the limb. The nerve may be severed, but the brain remembers the pain.

Deciding about Physical Treatments

Wait, if even cutting the nerve gives us only short-term results, how is it better than the other, less drastic treatments? And is it worthwhile to lose all feeling along that nerve for just short-term relief?

To put cutting the nerve into a proper context, taking homeopathics for the same back pain also gave short-term relief.[xvii] One treatment is an over-the-counter tube of homeopathic pellets costing around ten dollars with very low side effects. The other treatment is a surgical intervention costing thousands of dollars and with more serious side effects. But from what we currently know about chronic back pain, the amount of relief offered by the two options appears to be about the same over the long-term.

So, before you begin demanding opiates for pain (short-term relief) or consider expensive medical drugs or surgical procedures (short-term relief) or anything else (short-term relief) consider the reality that we have very little objective, comparable evidence about how well any of these treatments really work.

Remember, even if you read about a miracle pill tomorrow, there's still the issue of having no standard way to measure how well it works compared to other treatments.

A patient should consider the cost and danger of each intervention, deciding based on the reality that all of these interventions are unlikely to provide long term relief. Comparing short-term relief options realistically may mean putting off surgery or nerve cutting until after all other options are exhausted.

But we also know that, if even cutting the nerve itself doesn't provide everyone with long-term relief, perhaps it's time to look at other possibilities. Don't despair - there are other options to consider.

5 IT'S ALL IN YOUR MIND?

Before you slam down the book in disgust, I'm not going to tell you to "just use your willpower to overcome your repressed emotions manifesting as pain." That's the other side of chronic back pain treatment, and smacks to me of the belief that we create our reality entirely with our minds. Anyone who believes that we truly create our reality should close their eyes and use the force to ride a bicycle, or try to walk on water. Yes, I've tried both. One resulted in a crash with a guardrail, and the other resulted in a dunk in the lake. (In my defense, I was eight at the time and had just watched Star Wars).

While we all know that the mind affects pain, the idea that you can simply tell yourself to be well works only some of the time.[xviii] But we're missing the mark if we divide the mind and the body in our exploration of chronic back pain. We need to start looking at how much the mind affects the pain. Bear with me as we explore this side of things.

The Subjective Sense Of Pain

The sensation of pain is subjective, meaning that the pain you feel and how much it bothers you is largely determined by your attitude toward it. Take the example of a slight pinch on your arm. If you look down and see a grinning six-year-old, it's likely that the pain will be minimal. But if you look down and see a hairy spider or a small poisonous snake biting your arm, your reaction will be very different. The pain sensation is the same; it is the context that changes how much pain you feel.

Because pain varies with context, it can be changed by any number of factors. What you've been told by your doctor about the pain really matters. Is that agony in your belly just gas or a possible tumor? The story you tell yourself about the pain (it will pass vs. it will kill me) will modify the pain you feel.

But the variation in pain sensation goes beyond both the pain itself and what you think is causing the injury. A number of other factors may be involved. To give some examples, the pain can fluctuate depending on how well your day is going. How much pain you feel can be influenced by how well you like your doctor. (Is he a cutie or a pain in your butt?) Some back surgeons have started screening patients for depression because how depressed a patient is may actually determine how successful a surgery is at relieving back pain.[xix] Wanting to have better outcomes, a surgeon might refer a patient to therapy first. The therapy for depression alone may help your experience of back pain even without the surgery. [xx]

These are measurable changes. They can be so significant that they can mask how well or how poorly a pain drug is helping you. In other words, spending quality time with a doctor you like who tells you an optimistic story about your future just might be as effective for your pain as a prescription for yet another drug. (But get the prescription, just in case).

Physical Pain Causes An Emotional Response

We are all familiar with shifting from physical pain into emotional distress due to our internal stories. Nothing could be more straightforward. I bang my shoulder and I immediately begin the cycle of blaming myself or something (or someone) else for my pain. A variety of catastrophic events may pass before my eyes.

My shoulder being broken, maybe getting infected. I might see myself without an arm in a brief flash of paranoia. Usually this is followed by a prayer, often nonverbal. A deal is made. "I'll be good to my shoulder if it'll be fine, just this once. Come on, shoulder, give me a chance. I'll make it up to you. I need you shoulder. You're an essential part of the body team. I can't do it without you."

All this is done in less than a minute. The extent of the emotional response may end shortly afterward when I realize my shoulder is O.K., promptly forget it, and go about my business. Maybe later on I notice a bruise or something.

Physical Pain Can Create Habitual Response

But if I've really done a number on the shoulder, I may spend an hour or more complaining and cajoling my injury to go away. My day will be profoundly affected. The shoulder might heal slowly, lingering for weeks, possibly creating a new set of habitual responses as I favor it and use my other arm.

Even when the shoulder heals, I will likely remember how I injured it. I may remember the feelings I had about the injury. My body may remember those feelings as being associated with tightening the muscles around the shoulder to protect it. If I'm not paying attention, every time I feel similar feelings my shoulder may tighten. The tightening of the shoulder may remind me of the past injury, triggering more of those feelings, and around we go in a dysfunctional loop.

Chronic Pain Can Rewire The Brain

None of this is speculation. We can see it happening in the brain. Chronic pain actually alters the brain. Brain cells are lost and remapped in specific areas for each different type of chronic pain. Each individual has a unique response to pain based on how they deal with it. But there is an overlap in the base of the brain that gives a unique "signature" to the brains of all chronic pain sufferers. [xxi]

In the brain, sensing pain, thinking about pain, and reacting to pain all happen at the same time. Thinking about a pain can cause the body to re-experience it as if it is happening again. A person can also sense and react to pain without thinking about it. Think of the last time you touched a hot stove. You didn't pause to ponder if you should move your hand. Pain can cause a reflex reaction, like when the knee jerks up when tapped. These reflexive responses may take place anywhere in the body including the back without the conscious involvement of the brain.[xxii]

The Conscious Vs. Unconscious Pain Responses

Just like our physical reactions, we may not be able to control our emotional reactions to pain. The mind relies on the conscious, thinking brain to block the strong feelings coming up from the lower, unconscious parts of the brain.[xxiii] It's the process we call willpower, the reason we don't eat every dessert we see or blurt out all the things we'd like to say.

We "think twice," first with our lower brain and again with our upper brain, which results in turning down the dessert or holding our tongue. It works really well when the brain is dealing with something outside the body.

But chronic pain coming up from the lower brain doesn't go away just because the thinking upper brain tells it to be quiet. The emotional response to chronic pain appears in both sides of the brain. So while the conscious mind is calming emotions about an injury on one side of the body, it's not paying attention to the other side. The other side of the body is also reacting to the pain, but only unconsciously in the lower brain.[xxiv] So the unconscious lower brain on the uninjured side of the body is free to connect the physical pain to anything it likes: your emotional state, moving that part of the body in the future, being in the same space you were injured, or finding yourself in a similar situation. Without any conscious thought, you can create a repetitive, habitual response.[xxv]

Think of this repetitive back response like the story of Pavlov's dogs. Pavlov would ring a bell to bring his dogs in to dinner. After a time, the dogs would begin to drool just because Pavlov rang the bell. The bell, which had nothing to do with food, became a habitual, reflexive trigger. In the same way, emotions or thoughts that have nothing to do with an original back injury can cause habitual, reflexive back pain.

We can test whether people are aware of the back tension that could create habitual chronic pain. In a study of back surgery patients, about half the patients said they had anxiety before the operation. When researchers tested their backs for tension, these patients had areas of tension in the muscles on both sides of their spines. If you asked those patients if they were tense, they would know that they were, and their thinking brain could help them relax. But almost half of patients said they had no anxiety; they thought they were relaxed before the operation. When researchers checked their backs, these "calm" patients still had the same areas of tension in their backs. In other words, even those patients who were not consciously aware of it experienced "back anxiety." For some of those unaware patients, chronic back pain after the surgery may occur. But if you told them the pain was associated with anxiety about the surgery and that their backs tensed whenever they talked about the surgery, that might come as a complete surprise.[xxvi]

Within modern medicine, emotions like anxiety are often dealt with by means of drugs. Drugs make the brain happy, so the rest of the body shouldn't mind. But unconscious body responses are also taking place. Since drugs primarily act in the brain without relaxing the body, the body continues to experience the effects of the emotions in the back. But the brain on medication now thinks it isn't troubled by those emotions. So there's no reason for a person on anxiety medication to suspect any relationship between a major stress and a sudden back spasm.

We're not saying that the mind is a cure-all, either. But people in chronic pain can have significant benefit from "talking about it" (cognitive behavioral therapy).[xxvii] Studies of talk therapy for back pain show short-term relief. Which puts "talking about it" at roughly the same place as any other intervention, including back surgery or cutting the nerve.

Physical To Mental: A Personal Story

Recently I got to experience a direct body-to-mind back pain connection that initially felt entirely physical. I had begun a new yoga routine, and like all weekend warriors I decided that more is better. Afterward, I was driving my young son to camp about thirty minutes away. While in the car I began to experience ten out of ten pain in my right side while driving on the highway. For me that kind of pain comes on unexpectedly, is bad enough to make me grunt, and causes me to break out in a sweat. I know it's ten out of ten because it was the same level of pain that caused me to moan uncontrollably when I was recovering from surgery. It's that gut wrenching pain of a reawakening bowel, made worse by my need to focus on driving. To compensate, I started breathing faster, but stopped and held my breath when I felt my hands start to go numb (a likely indication that I was hyperventilating and could pass out).

Once I dropped off my son I tried to walk it off. Failing that, I drove back home to all my kit of supplies, but settled on spending a couple of hours in an Epsom salt bath and cussing myself out for overdoing the yoga.

Fast forward three days, and I still hadn't beaten this pain. (I did have periods of significant relief, and I made a plan to go into urgent/ER care if things didn't improve, but they did. I spent long periods without pain, then had it come back again when I overstretched) I tried everything in this book, except the mental connection. What mental connection? There was an overstretching of muscles; this wasn't some visitation by my guilt of ages past. But finally I was up at three a.m. and decided to just ride it out rather than haul myself up for another round of baths or exercises.

As I lay in pain, every single small muscle in my right hip area flared. Rather than fight them, I thanked them for trying to keep me from being an idiot. After all, they were the ones who'd had to keep my hip in place when the big muscles failed them. Each muscle told me I was an idiot, I thanked them, and they quieted down. Two hours later, I was pain-free. It did reflare when I ran four miles and then decided to play Hercules with the grocery bags, but another round of baths and apologies seemed to help. I also found a connection to an ancient guilt and let that go. In addition, I used a sulphur homeopathic, Tiger's balm, exercises, baths, stretches, prayer, and a lot of cursing. All of those may have helped some. But the major change was lying down and mentally acknowledging my stupidity. So even a purely physical pain may be addressed mentally, and I'm still learning how to deal with my own back pain even as I write this book.

6 FROM MASSAGE TO REALIZATION

If the mind is part of the issue, and the physical back is part of the issue, what about combining physical release with mental release? The combination, which is viewed by the medical field as "multi-disciplinary" because it combines areas of psychology with physical therapy, outperforms physical treatments alone. [xxviii]

While any physical treatment could include emotional work, most treatments are too short. Others are not conducive to talking freely because you're in a group setting. The exception may be massage or bodywork, which is normally done privately for an extended period. My own discoveries (which were really re-discoveries of the work of others) only happened because I use bodywork and talk with my patients during visits.

I also explore new possibilities with my patients, which doesn't often happen when giving a standard massage. The willingness to explore new directions, to try and fail, are essential in a good doctor/patient relationship.

Let me go through my own experience and training to give readers a sense of what to look for in a practitioner of bodywork, and to explain how I came to begin mapping the back for habitual responses (explained in detail in the next chapter).

Swedish Massage

When I first began doing bodywork training, I followed the standard Swedish massage model. A standard set of movements applies to all patients. The varying of the force of the techniques is based on patient preferences. But the standard model could be diagrammed out, and a person could create a "perfect" massage by dividing the time allowed evenly between body parts. It is possible to be a massage therapist for an entire career giving one standard massage, mechanically going through the motions based on a script rather than on the person involved.

I suppose I was already "ruined" for this model because

I had been giving massages without training from the time I was a child. Since I'd never learned the "right way" to do it, I would vary my technique greatly based on the person, the situation, and the amount of time available. My college classmates would seek me out to get massages on their shoulders and upper backs after long hours of studying. But I was only massaging and we rarely discussed anything emotional at the same time.

Naturopathic Doctor (N.D.) Training

During my massage training in class and clinic, I would get scolded for not following the standard model provided. It just "felt" like one area needed more work, while another was relatively calm. But I followed the standard protocols to get my grade, and kept giving my own kind of massage between classes to classmates.

The majority of my fellow N.D.s moved away from bodywork techniques as they began medical practice, and those that do bodywork tend toward the lighter energetic work rather than interacting deeply with muscles. So I had virtually no N.D. mentors who could teach me different methods of massage as I moved into my own practice. I had to seek teachers from other fields.

What Makes A Quality Massage?

In my experience the difference between a reasonably good massage and an excellent massage is the intent and focus of the practitioner. A poor technique can be applied to great effect by someone who is working silently on the body while consciously holding his or her patient in a space of non-judgmental positive regard. Excellent technique is wasted when the practitioner is burdened down by other concerns. When I've gotten these kinds of massages, I've just wanted to say: "if you really don't want to be here, do yourself and me a favor and reschedule."

The way I think about a bad massage is that it's like giving someone dirty water. Clean water, or clean intent, is action given freely with complete focus. If a masseuse cannot give without resenting the client, then they should cut back their hours or raise their rates until they don't resent them. It is fine to be compensated, and it is dirty water (not their best work) if they aren't able to be present.

But being present means listening, paying attention to what the client's body is telling your hands, and asking questions as you go. That's why, unlike most massage therapists, I talk to patients while I work. Without the combination of bodywork and talking I would never have made connections between specific emotional states and specific back pains.

Discovering Connections

When I started doing massage in clinic, a different picture emerged of what worked instead of a standard massage.

I remember working on two recent divorcees, one after the other, each with muscle tension between their shoulder blades. I would move away to complete my massage protocol, but the women would ask for me to work more on that mid-back area. Even after an hour of massage, they would both say that the pain was only improved.

Let's call the two divorcees Sue and Barbara for now. Sue and Barbara had very different jobs and activities. Barbara was an athlete who traveled for work. Sue was a desk worker who rarely took a walk. So the pain pattern matching for the two of them didn't make sense. Why would two different people have such similar pain? I questioned them extensively on habits or exercise routines, but nothing really seemed probable as a cause. It was frustrating to spend forty-five minutes releasing a small muscle group only to have it retighten within a minute or two.

Then one day Sue was talking about her ex-husband as part of the reason she couldn't stay on a good diet. He'd been unfaithful to her, and had tried to make her think she was irrational and jealous for a long time before he admitted the affair. Sue voiced the obvious: "I feel like he stabbed me in the back." When she voiced this insight, her back suddenly released under my fingers. As she discussed her husband's infidelity, her back retightened.

As chance would have it, the next day I saw Barbara. When I asked her how she felt about her ex-husband, her mid-back locked under my fingers. Barbara felt that she'd failed him, and he continued to play on her sense of failure to get her to continue to support him.

Here was the insight I'd been missing, which seems so obvious. A patient's emotional reality profoundly affects her back. We hold tension for physical issues, but we can also hold that same tension for emotional issues. The mind/body connection here is direct and measurable. (I tell patients I believe in the mind/body connection: it's called the neck.) We don't need extensive machines to measure what's happening; all we need is the patient and practitioner.

Over the last dozen years in practice I've worked with hundreds of backs. Many of them have muscular imbalance, but many have some level of emotional imbalance as well.

More interestingly, I consistently find a pattern that relates different parts of the back to different life issues. I did not come to this "map" of the back through a thought process, but by asking patient after patient about these issues and getting confirmation.

In one case I was absolutely certain I was wrong. The patient was extremely tight in the upper left shoulder, an area I had associated in previous patients with concerns about their parents. But surely a 78-year-old woman no longer had that concern? I very tentatively brought up my normal question about her parents' health, and the surprised patient explained she was indeed terribly concerned about her 95-year-old mother who still lived with her. So her back told me something I would never have thought of on my own.

Questioning The Map

Even after years of working with backs, I am very leery of claiming that a single map of the back is correct. But it can certainly be helpful when thinking about what stresses or concerns might be contributing to chronic back pain.

The focus must always be on the response, and the patient with the pain is the one who validates or invalidates any emotional involvement of the back. I have had several patients with intractable back pain who were unwilling to engage in any emotional discussion. We left it at that, despite the back bunching and jumping when they discussed their work. Since I live in a small community, I now know that one of these individuals was having an affair at work. But he couldn't get himself to recognize the contradiction between his work life and how he told others to live their lives. No matter what someone else's blind spots are, we must meet people where they are and help within the framework they provide.

Meeting People Where They Are

I don't start right in on chronic back pain being caused by emotional issues. The first step is to ask whether a recent trauma or other physical cause might have caused the pain. If patients have bruised themselves, it might take a few days to have the pain go away without dark emotional issues playing any role. A muscle tear might take several weeks, and a break in a bone may take several months. But any physical cause should have repaired itself completely within about six months. If the pain has continued unchanging for at least three months, it is officially recognized as chronic. At that point we know that something hasn't healed correctly, and we need more information as well as a different healing plan.

Even if something hasn't healed correctly and the pain seems odd, I don't immediately go with something emotional. Sometimes different muscles learn to spasm in defense of an injury, and forget to let go when it has healed. Moving out from the injury, I look for tendons, muscles, and joints that might have learned bad habits while compensating for the injured part. Letting these go while a person is relaxed and lying down should relieve the muscles, resetting them over a few sessions so that they can remember not to spasm in the future. It's this kind of muscle release that is most common from massage or from physical therapy treatments.

Only when the muscles have initially released and then retightened without any movement on the patient's part do I start getting suspicious that I'm dealing with some kind of habitual response. I suspect that muscle group has joined the "stress relocation" program of the body, placing any stress about an issue into that particular tissue. So that's when I start asking questions about the health of the family, stresses at work, and so on.

It can seem random, and it is a bit, until I get a telltale

twinge under my fingers. Alcoholic uncle? Back spasm. "Tell me more about this uncle?" Pretty soon I know exactly what's triggering the spasm - what line of mental reasoning is causing the tension. If your alcoholic uncle is coming to visit and your back suddenly spasms "for no reason," trust me, there's a reason.

By the time someone finds me and comes to my table, they have seen, on average, five other practitioners. They've seen their original doctor, a surgeon, a pain specialist, a physical therapist, a chiropractor, and someone else. All of these smart people have already had a chance to find whatever is wrong. My assumption is that all of them have done their work correctly and that there isn't anything they can do to give long term relief. So I don't waste my appointments repeating all the exhaustive testing that has already been done. That frees me up to explore what hasn't yet been done, which is trying to connect the dots between this pain and the other aspects of the person's life.

7 MAPPING THE BACK

We're all individuals, so please know that your individual results matter far more than my generalized guidelines. I only share my experience in the hope that it makes it easier for you to locate and recognize if your emotional life is contributing to your pain. You can take this information to your favorite doctor, counselor, or body worker and work together to resolve it.

The General Terrain of the Back

In my experience, the left side of the back represents the past. It is full of guilt and unresolved past emotional conflicts. Old responsibilities mount up, carried around in the tension between small and big muscle groups. If you've taken something on, it's sitting in your left back.

On the right side of the back, we have the future. Not a happy future, but a future of fear. All the things that could happen, to you, your loved ones, even the world itself, can get mapped out in your right back. In an election year I see a lot of back pain, mostly in the lower right side where our fear for the future of the world tends to park itself. But we hardly need a reason, as the unreasoning fear of the future can strike at any point.

I've also noticed that issues in the back tend to go from more general in the lower back to very specific in the upper back. Your general responsibilities to your fellow man and your concerns for the world would be in the lower back, while your guilt about missing a favorite aunt's birthday would be much higher up.

As we move across the back, guilt and unresolved emotions from the left side can lead to fear for the future on the right. These can move back and forth, as they often frustratingly do. My usual response to patients unable to let go of a particular concern, after I've chased it back and forth a few times, is that I don't mind if they worry all the time. But how is keeping their back tight going to help the issue? Usually they acknowledge that holding their back tight to the point of agony isn't likely to help, and that can finally ease the tension.

After years of doing backs, I can usually predict by

talking to patients where their issues are likely to lie. If a person is consumed by responsibilities, usually I check their left side even if the acute issue is on the right. But if they are facing some major life change, I will check the right side even if the issue they came in for is on the left. It takes only a moment to check, and doing so has rewarded me time and again with a true source of long-term relief.

Of course, individuals will confound simplicity by having a range of emotions play out in a dance. A problem with authority (left upper) and difficulty with one's children (left middle) will play out as fear of difficulty with a new partner (upper right). A practitioner must follow the tension and see where it leads, rather than assuming any theory will always be correct. But I get ahead of myself. Let's go through the different areas of the back, starting in the lower right and making a circle counter-clockwise.

Lower Right Back: "The Sky Is Falling"

The lower right back is where we go global with our fear. One of the best ways I can help someone with a lower right back spasm that has an emotional trigger is to tell them to take a news break. Stop filling their heads with some atrocity halfway around the world, and see if the tension eases.

Usually the lower right side is worst in people who are in the helping professions. They may wear their hearts on their sleeves, or be quiet, but they truly care and want to help. Somehow, through trauma or coincidence, they've learned to associate helping the world with holding lots of tension in their lower right back. When I point this out, usually the back releases · only to be back in a moment because they haven't fixed all of the world's problems yet. Lower right pain is easy to ease, but hard to keep gone. It requires a person to consciously shift how they are approaching their concerns for the planet or society. But doing that can lead to lasting pain relief.

An example of the lower right back pain is Carl (none of the examples use patients' real names and I have combined several patients in some examples). A bicyclist, Carl complained of right hip pain. After examining his hip and back, I released all the muscles and helped him correct his alignment. But as we finished we chatted about politics and Carl's pain came back as a sudden spasm. Since I had time, we worked again through his spasm and found three small muscles in his right hip. Each of these muscles really didn't like a particular politician. Invoking that politician's name could cause the spasm to recur. So we laughingly had to do a bit of an "exorcism" to allow this politician to stop being a pain in Carl's bottom. I also counseled Carl to turn off his car radio to and from work. We figured out he was resting his entire body weight on that right hip as he drove. So all the tension he felt about the news was going directly to the outer right hip.

Middle Right Back: "My Family Is Coming To Stay"

My patients say they love their family equally, but it's fairly easy for me to tell what the pecking order is in their extended family based on who's coming for dinner and how tense the patient gets.

Sometimes there's a favorite relative, but usually the tension of the middle back rises up in an unconscious ranking of who is emotionally closest to the patient. The lower middle starts with distant relatives near the bottom and ranges to one's children nearer the top. By the time we reach the shoulder blade on the right side we've moved from a person's family into the person's relationship with a spouse/lover/partner. Occasionally a person may have placed their work here, which tells you a lot about how much it matters to them (and how much they need to get out more).

Finding out which relative and situation is causing the spasm can be an "Aha!" moment for patients. Sometimes they've known all along on some level, but sometimes it's a complete surprise. It's as if their back has been telling them they aren't comfortable with some situation, but their conscious mind has been pretending it didn't matter. Shifting from "sucking it up" to "rocking the boat" can be all that is needed to gradually let this pain go.

An example of middle right back pain is Sara. She worked as part of a medical team so was very knowledgeable and gave me a sheaf of medical records.

It took me a while to figure out what was wrong with Sara. She presented with what she thought was physical pain, pain that had resisted decades of treatment but which wasn't quite bad enough for surgery (she had a "perfect back" X-ray).

Family issues didn't seem to bother Sara. She had problems with her extended family, but that didn't cause her back spasms. When she did physical labor, things sometimes got worse but sometimes didn't bother her.

The breakthrough happened on a day when one of Sara's co-workers messed up. She called me for an appointment, and on the table she wouldn't stop talking about the screw up at work. Meanwhile, I was releasing and re-releasing the same area of her right back. Finally, I started talking to her about how one of her co-workers messing up didn't reflect poorly on her. Her back gradually released as we talked about her work ethic and how unlike this co-worker she was.

In Sara's case, she had placed her co-workers on the same level as close family in her right back. Their work failures impacted her with fear the same way a child's health issues might affect most people.

Because of the nature of our relationship, I never brought this up directly with Sara. We never discussed emotions or religion. But I reassured her about her work ethic, and her decades of pain gradually eased to nothing. We were able to stop seeing each other. Now she sees a massage therapist occasionally. I think Sara suspects I did something more for her, but she's happy to leave it at a comment about "magic fingers."

Upper Right Back: "God, My Boss, and/or My Parents Are Angry."

As we start into the upper back, authority plays a huge role. It's almost like we all learn to tense our shoulders when we get scolded as children, and never forget it as adults. The fear of that authority and what it might do, whether it is a boss, a parent, an abusive spouse, or even God, settles in the upper right back.

I've often seen the crossover between fear of God's wrath as an adult and a remembrance of fear of a parent's wrath at some time in the past. These don't get separated cleanly, so a person may be afraid they can't live up to some expectation that they assign to God but which really comes directly from something a parent told them decades before.

Oddly enough, it doesn't have to be fear of God or their parents, it may be fear for God or their parents. If a person is concerned about their church or an ailing parent, their upper back can be tensed right up to the jawline. Holding that tension can feel like the best way for the patient to protect the parent, even when it makes no sense.

To really add to the tension, a person may feel the anger or fear and be unable to speak up about it. Feeling the bands of tension along the front of the neck, tightening down on the voice box, can be confirmation that this is the issue. (Or perhaps they're just holding back on telling you off for being a prying busybody.)

An example of upper right neck pain was Mary. She

came to me for help with her Rheumatoid Arthritis (RA) and we worked with some success on that issue. But Mary had neck pain so severe Remicaid and six methotrexate a day wouldn't touch it. She'd had multiple steroid injections into her neck that only helped a little with the pain.

Mary told me that overall her rheumatoid pain was a little better with the support we'd given her. She wondered if I could do something more about her neck pain.

When examining her upper back and neck, I realized very quickly that nothing I was doing was helping. As I continued to explore her neck muscles, I asked her about her family. Mary winced in pain. Another question, another wince. After the third question, she told me she wasn't sure what I was doing, but that it sure wasn't helping. I pointed out that I wasn't doing anything but asking about her family while barely touching her. She laughed and told me that her family was indeed a constant pain in the neck.

As soon as she acknowledged what was going on, her neck began to relax. I was able to release her entire neck and shoulder, which stayed relaxed until the next time her extended family decided to descend on her house. We learned to schedule her appointments for before family gatherings, so she could face everyone without pain. Yes, it would have been better to confront the issues with her family, but she wasn't of a generation to do that.

As Mary released her neck her overall pain improved. She had to decrease her pain medication for her RA six different times because it was now too strong.

While Mary does still have RA, the pain medication amount she was taking was primarily to deal with the uncontrolled neck and upper back pain and much less to do with her joint inflammation.

The Upper Left Back: "God's Hand On My Shoulder."

The simplest way to think about the left shoulder is that the heavy hand of authority has placed responsibility on us. It is more than we can bear, but we're unable to set it down. Individuals in our life who have authority over us (God, parents, our bosses) can set up a pattern of tension particular to this area.

It may seem that I move directly with patients from massage to Bible class, but I don't just start telling patients that they need work on their relationships with God. Let me go through how I approach this part of the back to give a sense of how I approach every area.

In the upper back I look for multiple layers of tension,

often centering around the trapezius' trigger points (where Spock applied his Vulcan nerve pinch) or stretching from the edge of the shoulder up to the neck. If you visualize a large left hand pressing down on your left shoulder, with resistant muscle tension pressing back upward, you can get a sense of what kind of tension can build up.

The uppermost layer of tension is generally physical in nature and can be massaged away without any emotional intervention. If it stays away and there are other focus areas, then you've released a great deal of the conscious pressure and can move on. But when it returns almost as soon as you've moved on, then you suspect an acute emotional issue relating to authority.

Usually I will massage an upper area two or three times into relaxation before I bring up anything verbally about the emotions. I generally find it most useful to begin with a question about work, followed by a question about the family or parents. In both cases, I pay more attention to the tension in the back than to the verbal reply. (Readers at home can try this for themselves by placing their own hand on the shoulder and asking questions.) Often tension in this area has been around for decades and may be completely unconscious. So the answer I often get verbally about any pain or issues with authority are, "No problems there. It's fine." Many people are completely unaware that their comment: "fine" is accompanied by a sudden shoulder spasm.

Once I bring the spasm to a patient's attention they may suddenly remember a recent issue with their work or family. Only after I get the second negative on both work and family despite a continuing underlying muscle spasm will I venture into religious topics. I explain that I've seen some patterns of tension in this area with patients who are having some spiritual difficulty. The term spiritual is less laden with baggage than religion. If I'm unsure, I will ask patients something like: "I don't want to offend you, so may I ask you about religious issues?" If it's OK, then I follow up with: "What religion are you?"

Once we've got the ball rolling in terms of a discussion, usually I will ask basic questions about religion. Generally patients are aware at this point of a possible conflict, and their shoulder will correspond to their insight by tightening like a board. Usually the conflict has not been dealt with on a conscious level, and the process of dealing with it consciously is enough to release it from the shoulder.

In the situation of a person denying concerns at the same time that the shoulder tightens, I again bring the person's awareness to the shoulder. We go through several rounds of testing the shoulder's response to different issues. They may consciously think they have no problem, but they can still feel their shoulders tightening. As soon as we confirm this, I ask them to consciously relax their shoulders. A fair number of people can accomplish a mental relaxation, and that will take us down another level of tension.

But a large subgroup of patients cannot consciously release their shoulders. Many actually tighten their shoulders rather than relaxing them. With these patients I ask them to do nothing, rather than "helping" me by tightening. Then I will passively move the shoulder around, often with a little random motion thrown in, to help the patient become aware of how involved his or her unconscious mind is in controlling the shoulder's movements.

Below the physical and the mental levels of tension is an emotional holding. As time permits, I may explore this layer while asking open-ended questions about how patients feel about their work, parents, or faith. (So, how do you feel about your work/parents/church?) I do not begin this at the end of a session, because if something breaks loose down at this level it generally takes a few minutes for patients to compose themselves. Once we've removed the mental blocks, the emotional release may come up at any time. Patients can be flooded with strong emotion they haven't felt in years, stored like a tension packet in their backs.

Since the upper shoulder often connects to our life purpose and our faith, I have often found patients at their most vulnerable here. A number of extremely negative statements about being a bad person, a bad child, or a poor worker may arise, blurted out by the patient. I often have to counter these with humor or with exaggeration because they are so horrible, then I respond with the opposite statement to whatever was said. Since in many cases I am really talking to a childhood belief that has never been fully examined, it is sometimes possible to offset the initial belief and replace it without a great deal of resistance.

Again, simply because at one point a person may have a religious conflict, I never assume that a set of tensions is emotional in nature before ruling out physical tensions. Fundamental existential questions may cause back tension, but so can chopping wood or lifting a box the wrong way.

An example of upper left back pain that moved up into the neck was Edmund. Ed came to me for digestive issues, but also had a diagnosis of epilepsy confirmed by EEG (a brain scan). He was taking medication that had the side effect of affecting his digestion. It also seemed unable to control seizure activity. Ed was barred from driving because of his seizures, so a friend brought him to every visit.

Sometimes people come to see me that I don't think I can help. When Ed came to see me I was pretty sure he'd gotten the wrong address. But he'd been through the specialists and medications, and he was hoping I had some miraculous trick up my sleeve to help control his seizures without his medication or at least control the side effects. I didn't, but he did have a sore neck. That I could help, and maybe make seeing me worthwhile. So I worked on his neck while we discussed dietary options for epilepsy.

His back was one spasm from top to bottom, and it didn't release with massage. So I worked just up on his neck. As I pressed just below his head, he told me a seizure was coming on. While not unexpected, this was alarming. I removed my hand and stood up to stabilize him during the seizure.

No, he told me, the seizure was subsiding. I returned to his neck, and again put my finger in the same place below his head. Again, he told me a seizure was coming on, and again I stood up.

We playing this game for a bit more before I came to the startling conclusion that his seizures were triggered by muscle tension throughout his back and extending up to his head.

In time, we were able to release his neck, and he reported far fewer seizures. Eventually, the seizures resolved entirely. We never openly discussed Ed's fear, his ongoing anger at the world, and his sense that he needed to fix the world. He wasn't open to that, but he sure liked my massages.

Despite being seizure-free for months, it took some time for Ed to get his medical doctors to recognize that he was no longer an at-risk driver. In their minds, the brain's activity had nothing to do with his neck or back. But after EEG retesting, they found he no longer had any sign of seizure activity. So now he can drive again.

Upper Middle Left : "Stabbed Me In The Back."

The region between the shoulder blade and the spine, originating around the rhomboids (where old movie villains would stab someone), is the area of tension I first noticed in divorcees. This area corresponds with intimate attacks on the heart from one's current or past partners. The betrayal here is acute and without respite. I've seen women constantly shift their shoulders, fidgeting to minimize the pain. They may consistently dislocate their own vertebrae or ribs, a situation made more likely by thin, tight bra straps below the area that act as back adjusting devices when put into constant play. One of my "amazing cures" is asking female patients to find bras with wider back straps.

Some patients are open about discussing their partners, while others tense up at the mention of their relationship.

The steps are straightforward: ask permission to discuss the situation, bring up open-ended questions while bringing the patient's attention to the area, and confirm that specific questions generate tension.

At this point it needs to be clear that my goal is ultimately a freed back, not complete mental wellness. While important, mental healing may be a much longer process than untying the unconscious connection between mental concerns and unconscious physical tension. When a situation seems too complex, I remind patients that they can think whatever they'd like. But could they please stop putting it into their backs? Usually this gets a chuckle and a release. For further mental care, I refer out to therapists.

Occasionally, a patient does not choose to have any

partner. In this situation, work can take the place of partnership and a patient can experience the same sort of betrayal and back tension from his or her workplace as she would from a partner. Men who have put work in that intimate location of the back often have broader issues stretching up to their necks. Perhaps for men the work/partner connection may be more intimately involved with his ability to deal with authority or his ability to speak freely at the workplace. For women, workplace betrayals can follow similar patterns to previous divorces and there can be several layers of tension.

An example of severe upper middle left back pain was Dorothy. Unlike some of my patients, Dorothy did not like to speak to me about her pain. She gave me a brief history and expected a physical solution.

Since Dorothy had seen many good practitioners without any results, I assumed that she didn't need anything extreme done and settled into doing what I could for her back tension. I worked on her back in silence until I realized that she was retightening as fast as I released. So I asked if she would mind if I "talked to her back."

It was a bit ridiculous, but I started telling the back what I was finding, how it made me think that these were issues about family, maybe an ex-husband. And the back responded, even though the patient did not.

As I became more familiar with the back's responses, I got better at guessing what was going on. Eventually we reached a point where Dorothy would talk to me freely because she said I knew everything anyway.

The end result wasn't perfection, but a shift from the habitual tightening, and the ability to discuss her previous alcohol abuse with her family. Her chronic pain resolved after that, and I've seen her for other issues.

Lower Left Mid-Back: "My Family Is A Pain In The...Back."

Family and friends make up the middle left back. With patients who are parents, this area is most often related to children. If someone has a large family, this area can include extended family, while with those isolated from family, this can be their peer group or even their coworkers. Rarely do I see back pain in child patients in this area, as their pain tends to fall higher into their shoulders.

Sometimes this area will be chronic and constant, but usually it flares up and fades. Asking questions about what's coming up for the family can elicit confessions of a party no one wants to go to, or a constant drag from a particular relative. These are family issues, and are not easily solved. But decoupling those concerns from the middle back, recognizing that Cousin Jimmie's rehab isn't going to be served by your painful back, can relieve a great deal of pain.

An example of middle left back pain was Deb. When I met Deb she was so out of it on pain medications that her family had decided she was incompetent to still live on her own. They were planning to sell her house and put her in a nursing home. In desperation, she had found me, and wanted to know if there was anything I could do.

Deb's back was relatively flexible except for a band across the middle. In my mental "back map" this corresponded to family, and indeed when she talked about family her back would spasm. Over our visits I got to the point that I could tell if her sister was bothering her, or if it was one of her children, all depending on which specific muscles were locked in her back.

Here we had a classic Catch-22. Deb had been caring for her family, putting them first, until her back pain gradually forced her to take pain medication. As she took more opiates, caring for her family became more difficult.

So Deb would worry more, which would tighten her back more, and she'd take more opiates.

Now we'd reached the point where Deb could no longer care for her family. Rather than caring for her in return, her family was planning to sell everything she owned and put her in a home. So Deb was worried and fearful for them and for herself, with good reason. But the opiates weren't solving the problem. They had become part of the problem.

As we talked about her options, Deb's back would relax. But the healing Deb needed was to stand up to her family. Having a little pain relief let her cut down on the opiates, which gave her a clearer head. Talking about her family's expectations and what was reasonable helped Deb focus on what she needed.

Once Deb was able to start setting reasonable boundaries with her family, her pain levels dropped. She kept her house, started a new business, and continues to live independently.

Lower Left Back: Carrying The World On Your Back.

Patients who watch the news too much should be aware that we keep everything when we take in the woes of the world. Everything we take in sits heavily on our lower back unless we consciously let it go. Any crisis, catastrophe, or horrible murder can sit here. For those who have pain higher up in their backs, it is likely that this area will also be involved to some extent. It's the dumping site for unnamed, undefined responsibility.

But because back pain only settles there when undefined and global, it can be easier to move this area by labeling and defining larger concerns. I get the sense that long neglected issues from the unconscious eventually find their way to the lower back, drizzling down from the mind and pooling at the end of the spinal cord. All it can take is a rolling up of the mental sleeves and a conscious sorting of the things that have settled down there to ease years of chronic back pain.

An example of lower left back pain was Marge. Marge came to me for help with family members and eventually came for herself when she couldn't walk. She cared for everyone: not just every human she knew, every animal she knew. Marge would lie awake worrying if her neighbor's cat was sick.

When working with Marge, we tried everything to get her to release her sense of responsibility for everyone and everything around her. Gradually, her pain eased as she was able to let go of some of her sense of responsiblity.

We did well until a family crisis took all her focus away from herself. Deb rapidly went from walking with a little discomfort to considering a wheelchair. She knew well that the stress of caring for others was worsening her condition. But Marge couldn't see how to stop caring and still be a good person.

Finally, Marge had surgery for her back and hip. While she recovered, the family crisis resolved itself without her involvement. She finally felt like she'd been given permission not to care as much. Since then she's been able to walk without pain. So sometimes surgery can be helpful for reasons besides just the physical.

Transitioning from the left to the right.

If the lower left back is involved, it is likely the lower right will have some involvement as well. But the right may be totally locked out even when the left is relatively calm and mobile. Patients may have had a relatively good life, be comfortable with their family and responsibilities, and still be terrified of losing it all. Their spouse may be exemplary, but they may hold a secret fear that the person will walk out tomorrow. Each aspect of the fear may trigger another aspect, so be very wary of right sided tension moving up or down rather than dissipating.

Putting it together.

That completes our circular tour of the back, starting and ending with the lower right. The whole map is a general guideline to give you a sense of what can hide in the back and where I have found it. While it can feel overwhelming, all that is necessary is an exploration of what affects the back. Unfortunately, a person in back pain is often reminded of that pain. Fortunately, those constant reminders rarely occur randomly. By expanding one's awareness from simply the physical (was I sitting wrong?) to the mental (do I hate that guy?) and the emotional (will she leave me?) a sufferer of chronic back pain may be able to find triggers and avoid them. In many cases, focusing on the triggers and working to resolve them can relieve long-standing back pain.

While patients can explore these possibilities with any practitioner, please work on finding practitioners who can help and are capable of recognizing that mental symptoms and physical symptoms do not exist in separate medical universes.

8 MAPPING YOUR BACK

If you've accepted that:

A) both the physical body and the mental/emotional state can affect back pain, and

B) that chronic pain may be altered by examining it and finding different ways of dealing with it.

Now it's time to take action.

Maybe the action you need to take is just a phone call to make an appointment. Ideally, you have in your community a body worker who is open to exploring different ways of releasing chronic pain. If they are just open to the idea, it can be enough to have someone work on the muscles involved while having an internal dialogue, asking yourself questions about what is going on.

But let's imagine that you have no one nearby. You've chosen a solitary life living in the arctic tundra or on a space station. How would you proceed to work on healing your back yourself?

The first thing to do is to break down the pain into its different parts.

Does a recent trauma account for the pain? That may be physical pain only, and respond well to physical treatments. If you've recently twisted an ankle and your back is sore from using crutches, no amount of soul searching is likely to be helpful until you heal enough from the trauma to walk on your own.

What worsens when you are stressed mentally? Likely there is a physical connection between that stress and that back pain. It's worthwhile to learn what causes that stress, what triggers it in you. Then remind yourself that tensing your back isn't helping your stress.

What gets worse when you are feeling strong emotions? These emotions are likely tied unconsciously to muscle tension. You'll want to start spotting the emotional change early on, and remind yourself that being angry or anxious doesn't have to play out in your back.

But say you know that stress or emotions are part of the problem but have no idea what might be causing it. Using my back map as a possible guideline, break down the mental and emotional possibilities by region.

Is it an upper right back pain? A lower left back pain? Does anything about my back map description trigger a memory or situation? When working with patients, I'm not fishing for just any association. Usually I want a strong response, an "Oh, yeah, that situation · ouch!" kind of reaction. If you can reach the area yourself, it should be easy enough to feel the physical response. Even if you can't reach the area, thinking hard and really visualizing yourself in that uncomfortable situation can be enough to make your back ache at that spot.

If you're still confused about how one part of the back connects to another, it can be helpful to get an anatomy book or look online for the muscle groups and layers in that area. Seeing how the muscles attach to the bones, how they are positioned on the back, can give you a better sense of why you hurt where you do and why it extends to where it does. Remember, it's not necessary to get a medical degree, you just want to understand your particular problem a bit better. If it's more confusing rather than helpful, don't spend the time trying to learn muscle groups.

Say you like looking at the muscles and want even more information about back pain. For those who want a broader sense of the back, looking up trigger points for the back can give you specific locations that massage therapists would push on to release the pain. These can be very helpful to know when you do get a chance to go for a massage, as it will focus the masseuse on those specific areas. [xxix]

Another way to get very specific would be to look at acupuncture charts and find the nearest acupuncture points. These points can be pressed on using the fingers (acupressure) and also give very specific directions to any masseuse.

Working with a Body Worker On Your Back.

Having a dialogue about your back pain while being worked on can be instructive. It isn't necessary for the massage therapist to initiate the conversation during a massage. Many of my patients start talking and don't stop on the table. So telling the massage therapist your troubles can be initiated by you, and you may gain insight into your pain simply by bringing things up.

For difficult issues, those chronic emotional problems that are hard to let go of but really need to be addressed (but not in your back), I have created a fictional character I often use. Meet the archangel Bruce, who is here to carry all your burdens and worries. Just for right now;

you can have them back anytime you'd like. But just for a moment during your massage, turn over those responsibilities and fears to Bruce. He doesn't mind, and he'll keep your burdens just as long as you let him.

The goal of any bodywork is to end the session feeling better rather than worse. It can be tempting to do more than you can handle, but be gentle with yourself. Don't plan to solve your back pain in a single session. Look for insight and improvement, then go home and work with the new information the massage gave you.

Home Work.

At home, there are any number of techniques to bring your attention to pain and shift it.

- Biofeedback machines can translate back tension into louder or softer static using sensor pads that can tell how tense you are.
- Tennis balls or other devices can give you pinpoint accuracy massaging certain back areas.
- A range of physical techniques from yoga to Feldenkreiss or Alexander Technique to Pilates can provide insight about your pain while also providing short-term relief of pain on their own.
- Simply sitting mindfully, listening to the body,

can also be helpful. Any number of meditation books and tapes are available to help with this process. One of the more famous is by Jon Kabat-Zinn, *Full Catastrophe Living*, which has a chapter on pain meditation.

These are ultimately not different treatments, they are different ways to get at the same treatment: awareness and reduction in pain by releasing and retraining the body.

If a person wants to explore further, the entire body can be examined for tension that corresponds to emotional or mental states. In my practice I have found that different points between the ribs on the chest can have specific grief memories attached to them. Other patients like to hide their tension in the soles of their feet. But the search for new aspects for dealing with pain should be enjoyable, not distracting or overwhelming. Using a single technique fully is far better than merely moving from one to the next.

Some techniques for muscle memory release can be taught easily (emotional freedom technique) while others (myofascial release) may take more time. I have found these useful for some patients who enjoyed them, but not for others. Sometimes practitioners of a single technique will forget that not all patients will benefit from any one technique. We don't all fit in the same pair of pants, so how likely is it that we would all benefit equally from any technique?

Five Mind Game RULES.

It's one thing to tell someone to be mindful of their pain, but it's another thing to help patients figure out how to do that. Just remember the five mind game RULES.

R.U.L.E.S.

Relaxing distant points. While sitting or lying quietly, focus on relaxing the distant parts of your body, working your way upward. (My toes are relaxed, my ankles are relaxed, etc.) In my practice I have found that asking patients to focus on relaxing a specific toe can often lead to the entire back releasing for a moment as they try to sort out how to relax just one distant part.

Understanding the cause. Sitting without thinking, and asking yourself the true cause of your pain can be either very helpful or very boring. But the hope is that you are on speaking terms with yourself and will get some ideas from your unconscious. These should be considered rather than ignored, regardless of how unreasonable they seem. It's an illusion to think that pain is always rational.

Listening rather than asking anything, focus on your breathing. Just listening to the body can be very informative. What are you aware of and where is it coming from? Does it change, or stay the same? In the momentary quiet, does the back protest or get quiet as well?

Exaggerating the tension. Rather than trying to relax, try to tense up. If you can do it without pain, tense every muscle in your body systematically. Then release it. Sometimes before going to sleep, doing this tightening and releasing three times can be very helpful.

Sitting with the pain. Focusing on the pain, think about what color it is, what sound it would make, how it appears to you if you try to visualize it. Watch the pain like an observer, seeing if it changes over time or stays the same. Does it expand or contract? Just stay with it, because clearly it wants your attention. Give it your undivided attention and see what happens. If nothing else, you're getting to know it better.

9 PUTTING IT INTO PRACTICE

Find neutral pelvis.

If you're in a back spasm, the very first thing to do is find the position of minimum pain, causing minimum spasm. In physical medicine circles, this is known as neutral pelvis. Taking a moment to shift around and find this position should be the first step in trying to deal with back pain.

But often in the middle of a spasm you're not thinking clearly and don't explore any little improvements you might make with the pain. A few patients have had their spasms resolve simply by finding neutral pelvis and relaxing into it. If nothing else, neutral pelvis lets you know how good it can get without any other intervention.

To systemically find neutral pelvis in a standing

position, gently shift your weight onto one leg. Lift and circle the other leg until you find the most comfortable position. Then shift the weight onto that leg and find the most comfortable position with the other. Once the legs are set, gently circle your pelvis to find the place where things hurt the least. Hold the pelvis in place and circle the mid-back to find the most comfortable position. Then, holding the back still, find the most comfortable position for the neck. By aligning your neck, mid-back, lower back, and legs, you can minimize the ongoing pain.

When sitting, finding neutral pelvis involves shifting the weight onto one buttock. Find a good position for the other and then shift the weight onto that buttock. Once both buttocks are as comfortable as they can be, shift to circling the pelvis. Follow by circling the mid-back and then the neck. The same exploration can be done in any position, starting from the weight-bearing areas and moving upward. Don't wait to be in agony, practice neutral pelvis in your daily life.

Neutral pelvis is one of dozens of techniques for dealing with physical pain. Rather than being overwhelmed, I would prefer readers take simple steps to helping relieve their pain.

Recognize, Realize, And Remedy: the three Rs.

To find your pain, remember the three Rs: recognize, realize, and remedy.

Recognizing your pain shouldn't be hard, but you need to define it clearly. Is it referred pain? (From your back up to your neck, for example?) Is it moveable pain or static pain? What are its best and worst hours? Describe the pain fully to yourself. What does it feel like? Is it sharp or dull, throbbing or aching? On a scale from one to ten, how bad and how mild does it get? What makes it worse, what makes it better? Do you like heat or cold on it? Really learn to recognize it.

Realizing your causes of pain. This involves watching the pain until you get some idea of what is underneath it. Maybe it really is a poorly healed bone. Or maybe it's because you hate meatloaf and yet always get served meatloaf by your uncaring mother-in-law. Watching is the only way to learn what is really going on.

Remedying your pain involves systematically going through possible treatments, keeping what is helping and discarding what isn't helpful. Patients can get trapped by themselves or a practitioner when they respond with fear toward change at this point. "It's not really helping, but it might get worse without it," means that you've decided to focus your energy on maintaining your pain level rather than getting better. There are ten thousand other treatments and a hundred thousand other practitioners. Move on.

Five Basic Treatments To Consider: M.O.T.H.S.

Not sure where to move on to? Remember five basic treatments. Of course there are dozens more, I just want to be sure that you've at least covered your bases before you settle for some treatment that isn't really working for you.

Massage

Massage is my first preference. Massage therapists are the most likely to be generous with their time (you can pay more for another hour · try doing that with your primary care doc) and the most likely to be open to letting you spout off about your emotions while they fold you slowly into a pretzel.

They also come in a very wide variety of styles, so ask

questions and shop around. Also branch out from your comfort zone. I thought I wanted hard massage until someone gouged me so hard they put something out of place in my belly. It took me a while to fix that one, and I now go in for a much milder pummeling.

In our insurance-based world, massage therapists also tend to be a cash-based practice. So those of you without insurance (or with such high deductibles that it is basically the same as no insurance) won't have to pay an arm and a leg to fix your back.

Osteopaths

Most people with back pain will have gone to a chiropractor. But few people realize that chiropractic evolved from osteopathic treatments. Many osteopaths no longer do physical work and are basically interchangeable with M.D.s, but if you can find an osteopath who does Osteopathic Manipulative Therapy (OMT), in my experience they use a gentler range of stretching and shifting techniques that may provide different results from the traditional crunches done by many chiropractors (other chiropractors use gentler techniques as well, so ask around for referrals).

Osteopaths can also double as primary care doctors and

are covered by insurance, which makes the right osteopath one-stop shopping for many of your health care needs.

Tennis balls

Any ball will do, but tennis balls tend to be firm without causing agony. They are also cheap and easy to find. Taking the time every day to think about your pain while gently massaging it with a tennis ball between a chair and your back is a good practice. If your doctor agrees, gradually moving from a chair to lying on the floor with the tennis ball under your back can do wonders over time.

There's nothing magical about a tennis ball for focusing your weight on one problem area. In a pinch I've used tennis shoes, rolled towels, paperweights, and even golf balls (not for the faint of heart) to act as massage tools.

While playing with the tennis ball under your back while lying down is good, those wanting more may want to use gentle, systemic rotation rather than just rolling in the four directions. I like the work of Moshe Feldenkrais, who uses a clock rotation model and who's training for chronic back patients is as effective as attending Back School.[xxx] Rather than just moving up/down, left/right, focus on tilting gently toward each point on a clock. Imagine the clock is on the ground under the tennis ball, and tip your pelvis and lower back up to twelve o'clock, then slightly left and up to one o'clock, a little lower and more left to two o'clock, and so on.

By working through the clock face rather than just the four directions, I've found that smaller muscles that rarely get attention are released. If the tennis ball is too painful you can begin with lying down and trying gentle rotation of your pelvis or upper back in the twelve directions. Then add the tennis ball under the most resistant knots of pain. There are lots of online resources and videos that go into much greater depth on how to use Feldenkrais for each part of the body.[xxxi]

Hot water

Before we had hot running water in our homes, we appreciated it far more. My favorite story is of an older man, we'll call him Biff, who was in a car accident. He was T-boned from the side and shoved across four lanes of traffic. Biff had no broken bones, but his seatbelt had bruised him all along its length. He refused any painkillers because he didn't like them. When I met Biff he had recovered from his seat belt bruising with only one treatment: his trusty hot water bottle. I remembered Biff years later when I was recovering from my surgery. Nothing helped as much with pain as my hot water bottle (an ever-refilling version that probably cost thousands) on my belly.

If hot water doesn't help, sometimes cold will. If neither helps, maybe alternating them will. There is an entire medical branch using water, called hydrotherapy, that has many wonderful uses for common hot water. If water feels too messy, many people use heating packs filled with rice, and ice packs from the freezer. Alternating hot (two minutes) and cold (20 seconds) can act in the same way as a massage by moving blood in and out of a clenched area of spasm in your back.

Surgery

Isn't the point of this book to avoid surgery? No, we should avoid unnecessary surgery. Sometimes a surgical consult can save your life. I had one patient with chronic back pain that resisted all treatments. Finally I sent her off to a surgeon because it just didn't feel right. She turned out to have an extremely rare form of bone cancer that was completely and safely removed.

No, I'm not saying anyone else has that form of cancer.

But I will say that patients who have limped along for years have benefitted from surgery. Others have had surgery with no improvement. Still others have been made worse. The point isn't that surgery is a cure-all, but it's a treatment that someone with chronic pain should explore before relegating themselves to a life of pain.

10 TEN CHEAP BACK HELPERS

It's hard to remember in the midst of back pain that there are literally thousands of pain relieving options. Yes, most of them may not solve your pain, but you should never feel like you've run out of options to try. Since we have no definitive long-term solutions, it makes sense to work with options that are cheap and easy to do. So before you shell out international postage on that new yak butter and bear grease super secret back cure, have a look at these first.

1. A quick lower back fix: 5-5-5 rule

One of the most useful things I have done for patients

with back pain is teaching them the self-correcting technique I call 5-5-5. It mobilizes the hips and releases the pelvis, which are often locked in odd positions for patients in chronic pain. Freeing the hips often results in freeing all the way up the spine, relieving tension in areas that haven't moved in days.

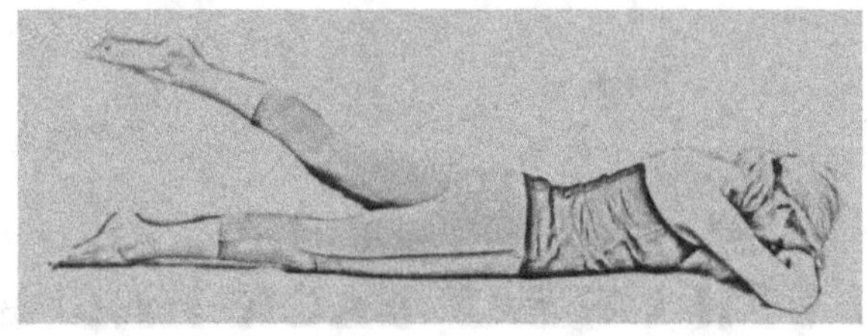

If you can ·WITHOUT PAIN · do the following.

Lie on your front on a bed or the floor. Lift one straight leg above and behind you, as high as is comfortable. Using small movements, circle it five times one direction, then five times the other direction. Finally, lift it as high as you can for five seconds before letting it down. Repeat the same process with the other leg. As long as there is no pain, doing this before bed can help chronic tensions ease through the night and may reset your chronic pain habit.

2. Ice

My patients may have seen several doctors but may not have not tried ice for their most recent back pain. They may have tried it once, or back in their childhood, but few people think to head to the freezer for back relief. If local ice doesn't help the pain, that's a clue that the pain may not be coming from that spot but may be referred down the nerve from higher up on your back. So don't just ice locally, ice higher or lower. When the area gets numb, you've had enough. Figure on about ten minutes. The minimum benefit you can get from ice is knowing that it doesn't help with the pain. Having that information can help your bodyworker look for other causes of pain besides local swelling.

3. Heat

If ice isn't helpful, heat may be. Think of ice as pushing away blood, heat as bringing blood to the area. So ice decreases inflammation, heat brings relaxation. The beauty of a hot water bottle or a controlled heating pad is that you can leave it on for an extended time. You can also use full body heat in either a sauna, steam room, or bath tub. Add a little epsom salts to the bath, and you may find other areas improving beyond your localized pain.

While many patients love it, some patients hate heat on the area. To me that's a huge clue that you may be dealing with chronic inflammation. Looking at the area may reveal redness and even old bruising, which has led some patients to suddenly remember an old trauma they had forgotten. But also be aware that this may reveal an underlying problem. Systemic conditions like anemia have also shown up in my practice as unexplained back pain and easy bruising.

4. Capsaicin

Want to shut down the pain but a little leery of surgery? The chemical found in cayenne pepper may help. A cayenne pepper or capsaicin (the Latin word for cayenne) cream will directly affect the nerve. It will cause a burning sensation, which exhausts the ability of that nerve to send out pain signals. No nerve signal means no pain in that area short term, until the capsaicin is depleted and the body gradually rebuilds its ability to signal pain, at which point patients can reapply the cayenne. It doesn't resolve the underlying issue, but it can give hours of relief. (Warning: Cayenne is a chemical that can cause burns, blistering, and will at least make your skin red. Use your common sense and check with a doctor before using it, especially on thin skin.)

Other creams use menthol or eucalyptus to do

somewhat the same thing. But cayenne is the most burning and the most depleting.

If cayenne doesn't work, guess what? You may not be experiencing local pain from that nerve. Some other nerve or muscle may be signalling from higher up or nearby, triggering the pain. Following up with some ice or heat nearby may give you a better sense of where the cayenne cream may be more useful.

5. Self-Massage

As I've said, I really like massage therapists as support for chronic back pain. But the best healing is done dealing with it daily, not twice a week. So massaging yourself gently for a few minutes a day can really make a difference in your long-term healing.

Where should you massage?

<u>A. Proximal to the area (upstream and down)</u>

Find yourself a massage tool, anything that will extend your reach. Something like a broom handle with a thick sock on its end can work if you don't have one of the many back massaging doodads. Don't limit yourself to the area of pain, move up above it and all around it. Be gentle, and don't injure yourself by doing too much.

B. On the opposite side

Sometimes an area is too tender, but massaging the matching area on the opposite side of your back can bring reflexive relaxation in the injured side. Think of it as using your new knowledge of unconscious habitual reaction for your benefit. Create a new daily habit of a few minutes of back relaxation.

C. Next to the spinal column

It can be hard to remember that the wiring for our bodies comes down from the head through the spine. If an area is tender, likely the area closer to the spine is also tender and that tension is causing worse pain. Massaging along the edge of the spine may be very tender but more effective than directly massaging the area itself.

D. On the feet

Yes, massaging your feet for back pain can feel crazy. But remember than all the nerves of the lower body have to pass up through the spine. These nerves are not plastic, they are porous like a garden hose with leaks. So massaging your feet and relieving tension there can release tension all the way up the spine and into your back. If you find any help from this, there are numerous reflexology charts that claim to show where the different organs are reflected in your back. But also be aware that the charts don't all agree so don't start relying on diagnosing yourself just by poking on your feet.

<u>E. On the ear</u>

Again, the pain is in your back, why massage your ear? In this case we have a whole tradition of ear acupuncture that claims the entire body is reflected in the ear. Since the ear is very sensitive and the muscles surrounding it affect the neck, think about massaging the ear as being relaxing down to the other end of the spine.

6) Prayer/Reiki

Many of you already pray for relief from back pain.

For those that don't, remember that handing over your stress to anyone, even momentarily, will relieve your habitual response. The act of asking for help sets off your unconscious mind to see if it can provide you with answers, and may lead to insight about something that is triggering, or may help with your pain. In other words, even if the Big Guy isn't listening, it's worthwhile to set yourself up internally with a clear goal about what you'd like to have change in your back.

For those of you who do pray, I have found that prayers commanding or directing the body are less helpful than more general requests for relief, resolution, and the wisdom to find a solution. In many cases patients' specific prayers for pain relief have been answered and their specific pain has resolved. But the actual source of the pain · the dislocated rib, problem with their seated posture, or habitual slouch · have not changed. So being open-ended with your prayers seems to lead to better outcomes than focusing only on what we currently know to be the problem.

Hands on Prayer

The sense of being touched in a caring manner brings all of us back to our upbringing, and sets off a series of relaxation responses that came before anything you've programmed your back to do in terms of habitual pain. Most religious traditions have some form of this hands on healing, and it's so effective for premature babies that hospitals will have volunteers lay hands on them.

Having someone care for you physically can be very helpful, but there can be benefits even if the person doesn't touch you. For the brain, physical touch is wonderful. But even visualizing someone helping you, trying to ease your pain, can be beneficial. The same parts of the brain light up whether or not someone is really there. So just having someone in the room thinking positively about your healing is likely to be of some benefit.

Within Christianity, the range of hands on healing

varies from Evangelical healings to Catholic healing masses.[xxxii] The Catholic church recognizes prayer as being an effective way to heal, while condemning some other healing traditions like Reiki. If you're unfamiliar with Reiki, it's the New Age version of laying on hands to heal. Practitioners may touch the patient lightly or hold their hands slightly away from the body as they send positive energy toward healing the patient.

A brief search shows a hands-on healing tradition in Islam, in Buddhism, and in Judaism. So regardless of your religious affiliation, it should be possible to find someone who will pray with you. For whatever reason, the laying on of hands is often considered more mystical than prayer as a healing resource.

<u>Distant Prayer</u>

Even if a loved one can't be in the room, it can be helpful to have them wish you well. Especially if you both take time out of your days to coordinate a time of caring. Most of us know that a phone call can benefit your mood, but even a shared silent time can help ease the tension of taking care of a problem all on your own.

Now we will leave the more esoteric and focus on things that your doctor can do for you that may not cost an arm and a leg but may really benefit your back.

7. Cortisone shots

A. Proximal - right next to the pain.

A doctor may suggest to you that a cortisone shot could fix the pain, and it might but not necessarily for the reason you've been given. Most shots are given directly at the site of the pain and the pain relief is usually immediate. The downside of the cortisone is that it blocks healing in the area as well as blocking inflammation.

B. Into nerve roots

Other doctors don't inject directly into your pain area but higher up along the nerve roots. Here they are doing the equivalent of a chemical nerve cutting, blocking the nerve's transmission of pain to your brain. But this is less effective than it should be, as the body rapidly finds other ways to get nerve sensation back to the area.

C. Saline injections may be as effective (nerve pressure)

When asked about why cortisone shots work, the prescribing doctors will wax lyrical about how cortisone reverses chronic inflammation. But many studies of the shots show that they are no more effective than a placebo saline injection. Not to say that a saline injection is truly a placebo. By injecting the area, you are resetting the habitual response of the area. As long as you mentally do not maintain the habit, either cortisone or saline can chemically interfere with an unconscious response. At this point no one has combined having someone do internal mental work with cortisone shots, but my suspicion is that they would become more effective.

8) TENS units

For those of you unfamiliar with the little Transcutaneous Electrical Nerve Stimulation (TENS) devices, they use between two and four little pads that attach with glue to either side of the painful area. The current they provide can cause the muscles to spasm, but is very mild and run on a nine volt battery. The purpose of the device is to allow your body to shock the muscles around the pain. In acute injuries they can help increase healing.

A. Muscle fatigue and natural opioid release

Constantly applying a non-painful shock to the pain area causes the muscles to become exhausted and to relax over time. As they tire, the muscles release endorphins, the body's own opioids, right at the location where their presence may do the most to reduce pain.

B. At nerve root to fatigue nerve pathway

Other doctors prescribe the TENS unit higher up on the body, along the nerve root to the area. Usually this is less effective, in part because the constant interference of the TENS locally with the body's habitual pain response may be the real reason that a TENS can provide longer lasting pain relief than just during and after its use. Think of a TENS as being a constant electrical reminder to rethink your habitual responses, and you can maximize its benefit.

A note about cost is relevant here, as I have seen TENS units sold for the cost of a lunch and for the cost of an iphone. Having used both, I would say that few patients benefit from the more expensive models. Unless you are planning to preprogram your own treatment plan, having a simpler model with several volume switches for intensity is all you'll ever need.

9) Anti-anxiety medication

A. Anticipatory pain relief

If stress makes your life more difficult and the pain of your back is contributing, it makes sense to look at medications that might help you tackle both issues. While the medication won't resolve either stress or pain, it will lessen the amount of "mind churning" you do that may contribute to both problems.

Many of my patients swallow Advil or other pain

medication and receive immediate relief, long before the drug has dissolved and entered their bloodstream. But those experiencing anxiety get almost instantaneous relief from just the process of opening the bottle. Becoming aware of when you experience relief and noticing that in connection to when the drug is likely to have been absorbed can help transfer the mind to relying on its own abilities rather than the drug itself.

B. Many natural options: valerian, hops, passion flower, etc.

While none of the natural remedies are as specific as the drugs for anxiety (I think of them as little monkeys in comparison to big gorillas) they have the advantage of not requiring a prescription and being available in teas. A range of different anxiety herbs can be found in almost any combination. If you're exploring this option, make sure you use a reputable company (I have several listed on my website under Fullscript. Anyone can sign up and go through the options.) because we lack oversight of herbal purity. The last thing you want to do is be anxious about what might be in your anxiety tea.

10) Muscle relaxants

One of the exercises I recommend to patients is to tense

every muscle in their bodies and release them three times before bed. For some this is a sufficient change from their naturally tensed state to fall asleep.

<u>A. Muscle clenching due to pain builds lactic acid=more pain</u>

The process of holding muscles tensed converts them from burning oxygen to anaerobic (holding your breath) muscle work. While this works short term, it causes the muscle to build up a waste product called lactic acid in the belly of the muscle. Over time, this lactic acid begins to burn like, well, acid in the muscle. It's what causes the burn from lifting weights or carrying boxes up stairs.

Long after we put down the weights or the boxes, habitual tension can continue and maintain a low level burn/pain in the muscle at all times. So a prescription muscle relaxant like Flexeril may release the muscles and allow your body to reset itself.

If a prescription doesn't inspire you, magnesium often works as well. To relax, the body needs to release its muscles. These muscles bind using calcium and release when there is enough magnesium available. So boosting your oral magnesium and taking long epsom salt baths can balance your system.

<u>B. Natural option Kava releases muscles and lowers anxiety.</u>

There's also a natural smooth muscle relaxant called kava kava. It was performing as well as prescription drugs for both muscle relaxation and anxiety when it was mistakenly tied to liver failure and pulled from the market in Europe. In the U.S., it was given a black box warning but the FDA left it on the shelves. After years of research, the Europeans quietly allowed kava kava back on the market because they realized there was no connection. But in the U.S. we still have the black box warning. So a relatively safe, useful muscle relaxant that also helps with anxiety is still treated with a lot more concern than it should be.

So there you have ten things that you might consider before having another back surgery or getting your nerves cut. As we end our time together, let's all step back to look at the bigger picture of back pain.

Beyond Back Pain: Triple A (Addressing the bigger issue, Action Steps, and Acceptance of yourself.)

Addressing the bigger issue: Back pain doesn't exist in a vacuum. Perhaps you've found some emotional or mental block that is a big factor. Or perhaps you've just realized that lugging cement isn't the greatest career choice as you get into your fifties. In either case, you need to take action.

Action steps: You need to break down what needs to happen, what changes need to be made, into the smallest steps possible. Why? Because humans are simple creatures and we like rewards and success to be easily possible. Otherwise we get discouraged. By giving yourself simple steps, you create a situation where you can succeed rather than fall down.

Acceptance of yourself. Even though you've taken the steps to try to succeed, the nature of human endeavor is two steps forward, one step back. (Sometimes it can be one step forward, two steps back.) The difference between improving and failing is the ability to accept that you aren't always going to be up and ready for the next step. Some days you just need to curl up with a book or binge watch something. The more OK you are with who you are and your own shortcomings, the more likely you are to be able to return sooner to the process of trying to improve your condition.

EPILOGUE

By the summer months, this book had been forgotten. I've been working on other books, with patients, and had other family crises. So this book had gone to the bottom of my "to-do" list. Then I woke up one morning, sat on a bad cushion for twenty minutes, and went to unload the dishwasher. As I stretched across the counter to put away a glass, I sneezed. My back spasmed in the middle, bad enough to lock me down. It left me holding my breath so I wouldn't fall because of the pain.

As always, hindsight is wonderful. If you know what you're looking for, you can always find an excuse for the spasm. I'd been driving for hours the preceding weekend, that darn cushion was unstable, and I was in an awkward position when I sneezed. More than enough to send me on a tour of the physical therapists, chiropractors, and massage therapists I know.

But I have a few tricks myself before I make the calls to my support team. I dropped to the floor, and began to do gentle clock rotations (the Moshé Feldenkrais technique where you move your back up toward one o'clock, then toward two o'clock, etc.) of my lower right hip. Think of it as pulling up, then up and slightly left, then up and a bit more left, etc. Once I'd eased the right hip spasm and found neutral pelvis (my position of minimum pain found by gentle exploration of what hurts more) I got up to go hang on a chin up bar. Taking the weight off my back and gently rotating it often relieves my pain.

Over the next ten minutes I worked through many of the techniques in this book, but nothing was working. The spasm continued. I recognized that nothing was helping. Then I asked what else could be causing my spasm. I realized that I'd been considering increasing my clinic hours, and that the area of the spasm coincided with an area of my middle right back that tightens when I'm concerned about patients.

While I'd been putting away the dishes I was feeling that responsibility, that I needed to do more for patients. I was worried that I wouldn't be able to take care of lots of new patients. Then my back spasm occurred, confirming my worst fears. Now I certainly couldn't see more patients.

Understanding the possible emotional trigger, I recognized the connection. Rather than arguing with myself as I had been doing, I accepted that it was a reasonable concern. I gave my back pain a place at the table, promising that I would reconsider if I felt stressed and that I would limit my practice to make sure my work was up to my standards.

Over the next ten minutes, the back spasm gradually eased. I still did some stretches and took care of myself, but the unbearable spasm was gone. As I write now, I'm not in pain. It's honestly hard to remember that I ever was.

The result of the back spasm was for me to return to this book because I realize others don't have the same tools that I do. I want to let you know that I don't have all the answers, that my back pain doesn't magically disappear forever. Life happens to us all. Just being able to recognize and realize all the causes of your pain can move you toward remedying it. If I can ease the pain of one of you, dear readers, then this book has been well worth writing. May you be pain free!

#####

ABOUT THE AUTHOR

Dr. Christopher Maloney went to Swarthmore College, Harvard University, and the National University of Natural Medicine. He practices in Maine, and has cut back his patient load since a bout with colon cancer in 2015. His hope is that this book is both helpful and useful to those in chronic pain.

If you found this book useful, please review it online and let other readers know they should spend their time reading it. Your short review and your two second rating matters far more than anything Dr. Maloney might say about his work. Pass on the help you experienced to others.

You can get other books from Dr. Maloney through online sources. His website, naturopathicmaine.com, has a listing of both nonfiction and fiction. You can also follow his twitter (naturopathealth), Quora (Christopher Maloney, ND) or blog posts (alternative holistic health answers). If you have concerns or suggestions for improving the book, please let him know by emailing docmaloneynd@gmail.com.

Thank you and best wishes to an end of your pain!

ENDNOTES

[i] Hestbaek L, Leboeuf-Yde C, Manniche C. Low back pain: what is the long-term course? A review of studies of general patient populations. European Spine Journal. 2003;12(2):149-165. doi:10.1007/s00586-002-0508-5.

[ii] Dawson EG, Kanim LE, Sra P, et al. Low back pain recollection versus concurrent accounts: outcomes analysis. Spine. 2002;27(9):984-93.

[iii] Haas M, Nyiendo J, Aickin M. One-year trend in pain and disability relief recall in acute and chronic ambulatory low back pain patients. Pain. 2002;95(1-2):83-91.

[iv] Qaseem A, Wilt IJ, Mclean RM, Forclea MA. Noninvasive Treatments for Acute, Subacute, and Chronic Low Back Pain: A Clinical Practice Guideline From the American College of Physicians. Ann Intern Med. 2017;

[v] Machado GC, Maher CG, Ferreira PH, Day RO, Pinheiro MB, Ferreira ML. Non-

steroidal anti-inflammatory drugs for spinal pain: a systematic review and meta-analysis. Ann Rheum Dis. 2017;76(7):1269-1278.

[vi] Haefeli M, Elfering A. Pain assessment. European Spine Journal. 2006;15(Suppl 1):S17-S24. doi:10.1007/s00586-005-1044-x.

[vii] Gianola S, Frigerio P, Agostini M, et al. Completeness of Outcomes Description Reported in Low Back Pain Rehabilitation Interventions: A Survey of 185 Randomized Trials. Physiotherapy Canada. 2016;68(3):267-274. doi:10.3138/ptc.2015-30.

[viii] Willems P. Decision making in surgical treatment of chronic low back pain: the performance of prognostic tests to select patients for lumbar spinal fusion. Acta Orthop Suppl. 2013;84(349):1-35.

[ix] Gugliotta M, Da costa BR, Dabis E, et al. Surgical versus conservative treatment for lumbar disc herniation: a prospective cohort study. BMJ Open. 2016;6(12):e012938. "spinal fusion should not be proposed as a standard treatment for chronic low back pain"

[x] Fernandez M, Ferreira ML, Refshauge KM, et al. Surgery or physical activity in the management of sciatica: a systematic review and meta-analysis. Eur Spine J. 2016;25(11):3495-351 "For disc herniation, no significant effect was shown for leg and back pain comparing surgery to physical activity."

[xi] Soliman J, Harvey A, Howes G, Seibly J, Dossey J, Nardone E. Limited microdiscectomy for lumbar disk herniation: a retrospective long-term outcome analysis. J Spinal Disord Tech. 2014;27(1):E8-E13.

[xii] Blanchette MA, Stochkendahl MJ, Borges da silva R, Boruff J, Harrison P, Bussières A. Effectiveness and Economic Evaluation of Chiropractic Care for the Treatment of Low Back Pain: A Systematic Review of Pragmatic Studies. PLoS ONE. 2016;11(8):e0160037.

[xiii] Hertzman-miller RP, Morgenstern H, Hurwitz EL, et al. Comparing the satisfaction of low back pain patients randomized to receive medical or chiropractic care: results from the UCLA low-back pain study. Am J Public Health. 2002;92(10):1628-33.

[xiv] Furlan AD, Brosseau L, Imamura M, Irvin E. Massage for low-back pain: a

systematic review within the framework of the Cochrane Collaboration Back Review Group. Spine. 2002;27(17):1896-910.

[xv] Bicket MC, Horowitz JM, Benzon HT, Cohen SP. Epidural injections in prevention of surgery for spinal pain: systematic review and meta-analysis of randomized controlled trials. Spine J. 2015;15(2):348-62.

[xvi] Maas ET, Ostelo RW, Niemisto L, et al. Radiofrequency denervation for chronic low back pain. Cochrane Database Syst Rev. 2015;(10):CD00

[xvii] Gmünder R, Kissling R. [The Efficacy of homeopathy in the treatment of chronic low back pain compared to standardized physiotherapy]. Z Orthop Ihre Grenzgeb. 2002;140(5):503-8.

[xviii] Schechter D, Smith AP, Beck J, Roach J, Karim R, Azen S. Outcomes of a mind-body treatment program for chronic back pain with no distinct structural pathology--a case series of patients diagnosed and treated as tension myositis syndrome. Altern Ther Health Med. 2007;13(5):26-3

[xix] Dorow M, Löbner M, Stein J, et al. Risk Factors for Postoperative Pain Intensity in Patients Undergoing Lumbar Disc Surgery: A Systematic Review. PLoS ONE. 2017;12(1):e0170303.

[xx] Richmond H, Hall AM, Copsey B, et al. The Effectiveness of Cognitive Behavioural Treatment for Non-Specific Low Back Pain: A Systematic Review and Meta-Analysis. PLoS ONE. 2015;10(8):e0134192.

[xxi] May A. [Chronic pain alters the structure of the brain]. Schmerz. 2009;23(6):569-75.

[xxii] Peyron R, Laurent B, García-larrea L. Functional imaging of brain responses to pain. A review and meta-analysis (2000). Neurophysiol Clin. 2000;30(5):263-88

[xxiii] Green MJ, Cahill CM, Malhi GS. The cognitive and neurophysiological basis of emotion dysregulation in bipolar disorder. J Affect Disord. 2007;103(1-3):29-42.

[xxiv] Garcia-larrea L, Peyron R. Motor cortex stimulation for neuropathic pain: From phenomenology to mechanisms. Neuroimage. 2007;37 Suppl 1:S71-9.

[xxv] Cheng JC, Erpelding N, Kucyi A, Desouza DD, Davis KD. Individual Differences in Temporal Summation of Pain Reflect Pronociceptive and Antinociceptive Brain Structure and Function. J Neurosci. 2015;35(26):9689-700

[xxvi] Esin RG, Danilov VI, Minkina ISh, Esin OR. [Failed back syndrome in patients after the surgery for compressive lumbosacral radiculopathy]. Zh Nevrol Psikhiatr Im S S Korsakova. 2009;109(11):37-41.

[xxvii] Schechter D, Smith AP, Beck J, Roach J, Karim R, Azen S. Outcomes of a mind-body treatment program for chronic back pain with no distinct structural pathology--a case series of patients diagnosed and treated as tension myositis syndrome. Altern Ther Health Med. 2007;13(5):26-35.

[xxviii] Kamper SJ, Apeldoorn AT, Chiarotto A, et al. Multidisciplinary biopsychosocial rehabilitation for chronic low back pain: Cochrane systematic review and meta-analysis. BMJ. 2015;350:h444.

[xxix] https://www.painscience.com/tutorials/trigger-points.php

[xxx] Paolucci T, Zangrando F, Iosa M, et al. Improved interoceptive awareness in chronic low back pain: a comparison of Back school versus Feldenkrais method. Disabil Rehabil. 2016;:1-8.

[xxxi] https://www.youtube.com/watch?v=IEoFeAGlaho

[xxxii] https://www.ewtn.com/library/Liturgy/zlitur276.HTM

9 781976 214974